Pain in Older People and People with Dementia: A practice guide

Dr William McClean with
Colm Cunningham

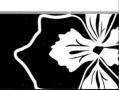

Dr William McClean:

Bill has worked as a consultant physician in geriatrics since 1985 following10 years as a consultant in general medicine. He has been based in Taree a regional town in New South Wales. This work has been in acute hospitals, rehabilitation and long term institutional care, as well as in the community. His research interests have been in clinical epidemiology and the application of these principles to pain management in people in longer term institutional care.

He has spent some time in consulting in Aged Care facilities in NSW assessing and advising on the pain management of the residents. At present he is medical director of the Rehabilitation and Assessment Unit at Wingham Hospital and Riverview Lodge, a unit for older people with dementia and special behavioural needs.

Colm Cunningham:

Colm Cunningham is Director of Operations at The Dementia Services Development Centre, University of Stirling. He has worked with Dr McClean to produce this new version of the practice guide and has undertaken a number of research projects relating to the issue of pain management in people with dementia.

Acknowledgments:

Dr Bill McClean has worked with The Dementia Services Development Centre on a number of projects to highlight the pain needs of people with dementia. In 1999 Dr McClean wrote, 'Practice Guide for Pain Management for People With Dementia in Institutional Care'. This new publication 'Pain in Older People and People with Dementia: An practice guide' is a revised version of this publication, containing additional materials to support practitioners in meeting the pain needs of older people and people with dementia.

The Dementia Services Development Centre is extremely grateful to Dr McClean for his work to produce this new publication and to the staff of Macmillan Cancer Relief, Jean Phillips of Strathcarron Hospice and Professor Bill MacLennan for their assistance with the original publication. Thank you also to Professor Jennifer Abbey for permission to reproduce the Abbey Pain Scale.

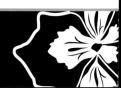

Contents

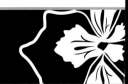

Introduction:

Pain affects a significant proportion of the older population and is often not recognised or effectively treated. A number of older people and people with dementia and may not be recognised or treated effectively. This practice guide has been written to aid staff in their understanding of pain and to consider ways to improve their individual and organisational approaches to the management of pain in older people and people with dementia.

This practice guide can be used in two ways:

> **A self study guide:** The reader is able to work through each section of the book undertaking the individual exercises within a chapter. The reader can draw further useful information by reading the 'Notes for Facilitators' after undertaking an exercise by referring to these in Chapter 5. The individual notes for facilitators is identified by **'NF'** followed by a reference number.

> **A facilitator training guide:** The practice guide is also designed to enable a facilitator to develop a series of individual education sessions or a study day. The individual exercises along with the 'Notes for Facilitators' are design to be used to guide staff through the stages of engaging with the issues of pain in older people and people with dementia. The materials used in this book can be reproduced by a facilitator for this purpose, but full reference must be given to the source materials. Copyright is only granted within this context.

It is important to note that despite the majority of research quoted within this guide being undertaken within a nursing context, similar studies within a non-nursing care home environment indicate that the issues raised are replicated within these settings.[1]

The practice guide is designed to enable staff to be better informed of the pain needs of older people and people with dementia and of strategies and approaches to support these needs. Clinical decisions about the pain management of a specific individual should be based on the advice of an appropriately authorised practitioner and not solely on the content of this guide.

---

[1] Cunningham C 2006, Determining whether to give pain relief to people with dementia: the impact of verbal and written communication on the decision to administer 'as required' analgesia to people with dementia in care homes Alzheimer's Care Quarterly 7(2) 95-103

1 What is the Problem?

Aim: To think about the issue of pain as a personal experience.

Contents

a): What is pain?

There are many ideas about "pain". We sometimes use the word rather loosely to mean anything we do not like. Sometimes you may hear people say about a person who has annoyed them, "She is a pain". Sometimes we also talk about "mental pain" when we mean great emotional distress. However, strict use of the word applies to a sensation of the body. In this guide we will be using the word "pain" in this restricted sense.

Our definition: Pain relates to a sensation of the body.

 1. Exercise: Self reflection

> **Think of a situation where you have felt pain. How would you describe it?**
> **Try and write in the space below what pain was for you.**

NF1

There are many definitions of pain and each one will reflect something of the person who is writing the definition. One well-used definition has been worked out by the International Association for the Study of Pain. It says that pain is an unpleasant sensory and emotional experience that we associate with tissue damage.

Other researchers on pain have proposed that pain involves three types of experience:

*   the actual sensation
*   the knowledge about the pain
*   the emotional aspect

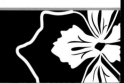

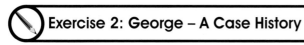

Think about the following story, and comment on the questions in the boxes:

NF2

——— 10 ———

George was 65 years old. He was not very physically active. One day he decided to do some gardening. He spent most of the morning digging and bending over weeding. That night he had a hot bath and went to bed. The following morning he had what he described as stiffness and soreness in his shoulders and his back. George commented to his wife, "I must have done some good exercise, because I'm aching in muscles I never knew that I owned."

> **1. What do you think George's emotional state was that morning when he commented to his wife about the aches in his muscles?**

NF3

George continued to have these aches in his muscles. The pains were no worse; they just persisted. Eventually after two weeks he went to his doctor who examined him, and ordered some blood tests and X-rays.

> **2. What do think George is feeling now?**

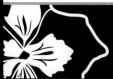

George went to the doctor to obtain the results of the tests. His doctor told him that one of the tests was abnormal and that George may have cancer of the prostate which may have spread to the bones.

3. What do you think George is feeling about the aches now? Do you think that they seem worse or better than when he first experienced them? Why?

More tests were ordered. When George went to the doctor for his report his wife went with him. They were very relieved to find out that the tests were clear and that the cause of the pains was a simple disease that could be treated with some physiotherapy, and that George should be free from symptoms in a couple of weeks' time.

4. Do you think that the pains worried George now? Why?

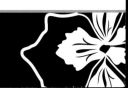

Although George's sensation of pain may not have increased at the time he was concerned about having cancer, the actual pain experience would have been more unpleasant. His knowledge led to a change in the emotional aspect of the pain.

Perhaps you can see how pain involves the actual sensation which may have certain characteristics of intensity, position etc. However, it has emotional meaning and it is also affected by what we know about the pain. The pain we experience is a complex combination of these three aspects: sensation, knowledge and emotion.

An older person or person with dementia may have long-term memories of childhood pain experiences which were very frightening. These memories may revive even in dementia to make the pain of late life much more distressing. How else may the progression of dementia interact with one or more of these three aspects of the pain experience?

Previous experience of pain can influence how a person reacts to pain. It can be helpful or make the experience more distressing. So memory of pain is important in the experience. When thinking about pain management in older people and people with dementia it is necessary to consider these aspects of pain: the sensation, and the knowledge and emotion associated with the pain.

 Exercise 3:

Imagine a young person who is a keen athlete, training for a marathon run. The process of training for such an event involves pain. Try to analyse the pain experience of training and running a marathon in terms of the:

- sensation
- knowledge
- emotion

b): Types of Pain

Doctors assessing pain have various ways of analysing pains based on what the person tells them. Many doctors use the following classification to think about pain:

1. **Acute Pain:** is defined as pain that is of relatively recent onset. It is a response to tissue injury. It resolves as tissue healing occurs. It generally lasts less than a month or so.

2. **Chronic Pain:** is said to exist if it persists for more than a month beyond the course of an acute illness or a reasonable time for healing to occur, if it is due to a chronic pathological process, or if it recurs at intervals for months or years.

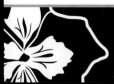

3. Chronic Malignant Pain: if a cancerous process is suspected to be the cause of the pain.

4. Chronic Non-Malignant Pain: if a cancer is not suspected as the cause of the pain. Chronic non-malignant pain is the most common pain among older people. It is often the most difficult to treat and causes a lot of disability.

Sometimes an injury may cause an acute pain and the pain may continue even after the injury has had time to heal. The actual cause of this is not fully understood, but continued chronic pain is not really known but the pain is very real and debilitating. It is generally called "Chronic Pain Syndrome". We will not be dealing further with this although we will be thinking about chronic pain arising from chronic disease processes. It is important to remember that pain may be present without an obvious cause.

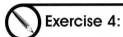 **Exercise 4:**

Classify these causes of pain into:

Acute   = A
Chronic Malignant   = CM
Chronic Non-Malignant   = CN

Burning a finger on a hot iron	
Osteoarthritis of the knee	
Heart attack (myocardial infarction)	
Peritonitis from perforated stomach ulcer	
Cancer of the breast Involving the vertebrae	
Osteoporotic fractures of the spine	
Pain after an attack of shingles	

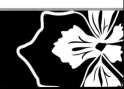

Note: Whatever the cause of pain, it is always real to the individual and makes us feel and behave in certain ways.

Burning a finger on a hot iron causes acute pain. Osteoarthritis of the knee causes chronic non-malignant pain. A heart attack and peritonitis cause acute pain. Cancer of the breast involving the vertebrae causes chronic malignant pain. Osteoporotic fractures of the spine cause acute pain which can become chronic non-malignant.

c): How Do we React to and Communicate about Pain?

Two useful terms are:

- pain threshold
- pain tolerance

Pain Threshold

When a stimulus, such as heat or pressure is applied to our skin, at first it may not be painful. As the temperature rises or the pressure increases, a point is reached when we think, "This is painful". That point is called the "pain threshold". It can be measured for any person or group of people, by gradually increasing a stimulus until pain is experienced.

Pain Tolerance

Pain tolerance is measured by the amount of time that a person can tolerate a certain pain level. (This is different from the medical use of the term which refers to the phenomenon whereby a patient gets used to pain-killing drugs (or several other drugs including tranquillisers and antidepressants) and requires ever-increasing doses to maintain the level of pain control).

Verbal Communication

As we found in Section 1, pain affects us differently according to the sensation, the knowledge and the emotions associated with the experience. How we react to any pain also depends on our culture and our previous experience. Studies have shown that various cultures deal with pain in different ways. Also, there can be differences between the ways that the older generation reacts to pain compared with younger people.

Although it is not wise to generalise too much, people from Southern Mediterranean cultures often deal with pain by sharing the experience. In contrast, Northern European culture tends to be less demonstrative and "keep a stiff upper lip". One should not make value judgements on either way of reacting to pain, but we should be aware that these differences might account for some of what we observe in the people we care for professionally. Many of the older

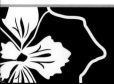

generation were brought up in a culture that encouraged stoicism and non-complaining. This can lead older people to under estimate their pain and this will lead professionals also to under estimate the significance of their patient's symptoms. Research in the USA and Europe has shown that, generally, professionals understate the pain that their patients/clients are experiencing. So to correct this, it is probably wise to over estimate, rather than play down the pain that the patient/client is experiencing.

 Exercise 5:

Place the following thirteen words in order of strength or severity. Do this initially without consulting any one else. If you can then ask someone else to do this exercise and then compare the two lists.

Paining, Aching, Hurting, Sore, Stinging, Tender, Excruciating, Agonising, Uncomfortable, Burning, Smarting, Niggling, Sensitive

Least severe

1
2
3
4
5
6
7
8
9
10
11
12
13

Most severe

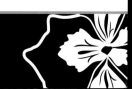

You may note that there are differences in the way that each person uses the language associated with pain. We must be aware that this fact is active in the way that people communicate their experience of pain. Our understanding of words may be different from that of the person we are caring for. The greater the age difference and the greater the cultural difference the more chance there is of misunderstanding. So it is important to delve deeper into what the person is saying about their pain experience, to ask more specific questions about their pain.

Non-verbal Communication

As well as verbal language that communicates to other people about our pain, body language and behaviour may tell other people that we are in pain. It is important for those who care for older people to be sensitive to body language and behaviour in assessing pain. It is also important to realise the limitations of body language and behaviour in this situation.

There is some evidence to suggest that verbal reports about pain are sampling different aspects of the pain experience than the non-verbal responses. This means that where possible any pain assessment should try to take into account both verbal and non-verbal information from the patient.

Acute Pain

When a person experiences acute pain, there are changes in that person which an observer can detect.

Physiological Changes

In severe acute pain, such as in a heart attack, the person may become very pale, and sweating may occur. The blood pressure may become lowered, and the person may faint, or vomiting may result. These are referred to as "physiological changes".

These physiological changes are sometimes less obvious in very old people and so they cannot always be relied on to indicate acute pain. For instance, in people over the age of 75 years the only sign of a heart attack may be the sudden onset of mental confusion.

Body Language

Body language is also an important clue to the presence of pain.

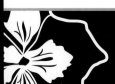

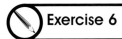

Try to match the following body language/behaviours with possible sites of pain:

a) Refuses to put weight on left lower limb
b) Spits out food when being fed
c) Lies with knees drawn up
d) Pulls away when right arm is touched
e) Hits out at the nurse when being turned in bed

Sore tooth   **Abdominal pain**   **Pain in shoulder**

Pain in left hip   **Pain in back**

You will notice that it is hard to distinguish between body language and behaviour. The one blends into the other.

NF16

Behaviour

The third way in which non-verbal communication occurs to express acute pain is through behaviour. Our behaviour is influenced when we have pain. At one level pain is often a reason for us being intolerant or cranky. It can make us restless, or cause us to change position or fidget. The same thing happens in older people or those with dementia. Other behaviours can be observed in people with pain.

Chronic Pain

When pain has been going on for a long time, that is when it has become chronic, the body's physiological reactions become "worn out" or blunted. This means that the usual pallor, sweating etc. do not occur. Thus, as a means of assessing whether or not pain is present, these observations are not helpful.

Certain behaviours may be helpful in confirming chronic pain to be present, but even here it may not be possible to detect any behaviour that we would typically associate with pain. It has been widely said that "pain is whatever the subject says it is". The patient is the expert on his or her own pain. With chronic pain the only evidence that may be present is the person's verbal report, and it is wise to believe that report.

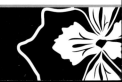

Exercise 7

Which of the following would you think are the consequences of suffering from chronic pain? Can you think of other possible consequences?

	Yes	No
Depression	❏	❏
Decreased socialisation	❏	❏
Sleep disturbance	❏	❏
Impaired mobilisation	❏	❏
Increased healthcare utilisation	❏	❏
Increased healthcare costs	❏	❏
Drug dependency	❏	❏
Suicide	❏	❏

In fact all of these are consequences of experiencing chronic pain.

NF17

Summary of this Chapter

This chapter has covered the following topics:

- Pain is an unpleasant experience which involves sensation, knowledge and emotion.
- Pain can be acute, with obvious physiological changes, or chronic without those same physiological changes. Chronic pain can be non-malignant or malignant.
- There are cultural differences in the way people deal with pain and express pain.
- Pain is expressed by verbal and non-verbal communication.
- Nonverbal communication involves physiological changes, body language and behavioural changes.
- Chronic pain has many social and health consequences.

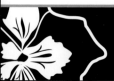

2 Older People in Pain

Aim: To think about the issue of pain experience in community settings, acute care wards and long-stay institutional care/care homes.

Contents

a) Older People Living in the Community

Surveys of older people living in the community indicate that at least 25-50% experience important pain problems. The main source of the pain is the joints and back.

When aged people are living in their own homes, they may have more control over the treatment of their pain. They have the choice of going to their medicine chest and finding a painkilling medication or applying heat to the area. They can make an appointment to consult their doctor and have the pain issue treated. Surveys have shown that 18% of older Americans are taking analgesic medications regularly. Of those, 63% have taken prescription pain medications for more than 6 months, and 45% of those taking pain medications regularly had seen more than three doctors about their pain in the previous five years. So pain among older people living in the community is a very significant problem. However, the choice to obtain treatment remains largely with the individual.

b) Older People in the Acute Hospital Ward

There is ample evidence that older people receive fewer post-operative pain medications than do younger adults. In fact, the older a patient is, the less likely that patient is to receive adequate analgesia.

If, in addition, patients have dementia, there is even greater probability that they will not receive adequate post-operative pain treatment. (One study showed that analgesic medication was administered to 67% of older people with normal cognition, compared with only 17% of those with dementia).

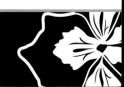

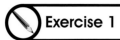 **Exercise 1**

> **What factors are operating to prevent adequate pain management in older people and those with dementia? Try to think of three.**
>
> 1
>
> 2
>
> 3

NF3

How do you think this trend could be reversed?

NF4

c) Older People in Care Homes

Studies have been done to determine the numbers of people who are in pain in long-term care. That is, the prevalence of pain has been measured in various ways. The prevalence of pain depends on how we measure "pain". If we are interested in pain at the time that the subject is being assessed or questioned, we will obtain a different result than if we ask about the subject's pain in the past day or week. If we record past pain as well as present pain, the prevalence figure will be higher. Some studies have found prevalence of pain in care homes to be as high as 80%. A survey that was conducted by the author of this workbook showed that 25% of residents who were able to communicate verbally were in pain at the time of interview; another 30% had pain at other times, giving 56% who had pain problems. In lower care facilities (with lower nursing needs) the proportion was even higher (63%).

 Exercise 2

> **What other factors will influence the prevalence of pain in any long-term facility?**

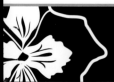

Among the factors you have thought about, the following may have occurred:

- The types of diseases suffered by the residents.
- The priority given by the staff and management, to treating pain.

One large American study of palliative treatment in care homes followed 13,625 patients with cancer from hospital to care homes. Four thousand and three reported daily pain. Older patients and those with dementia were less likely to receive adequate pain relief. About 26% of those in pain did not receive any analgesics, and a high proportion of them were over 85 years old. Other studies showed similar results for care home residents with chronic non-malignant pain.

People in care homes have sites of pain similar to those of people living in the community. The most prevalent pains are in the joints, limbs and the back. These pains are due most commonly to arthritis. It may be thought that we are dealing with mild pain among these old people. However, care home residents most commonly describe the pain they have as being severe, rather that moderate or mild. Even allowing for the fact that these studies have been carried out in the USA and Australia, this research shows that a lot can be done to improve the comfort of older people in care homes in any country.

Think of the older people that you care for. Do you think all those who need it are receiving adequate pain relief?

Dementia and Pain

There is ample evidence that those people with dementia, living in care homes, do not receive as much treatment for pain as those with normal cognition. In chapter 3 we will look at this fact in more detail.

d) Staff Awareness

Imagine a care home of 50 residents, of whom 35 are able to communicate verbally. Now imagine that 12 residents are in pain at a particular point of time. Guess how many of these people would be known to the nursing staff as having a pain problem?

(a) 12 (b) 10 (c) 8 (d) 6 (e) 4 (f) 2

The Australian study quoted above looked at the recording of pain in the nursing notes. There was agreement between what the patient said and the nursing notes in only 58% of cases. Let

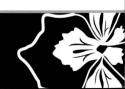

us apply this finding to the situation in the exercise above. It means that the nurses would be aware of the possibility of pain in about **7** of the residents who were in pain. The other **5** would suffer from pain without the nurses being aware of the possibility.

Pain recording in care homes will vary considerably, depending on the management's expectation and demands, the type of facility, and the experience and attitudes of the staff.

However, it is interesting to look at what nurses record in their notes each shift. This has been done; and the ten categories of information placed in order. The following table shows the categories chosen after the nursing notes had been examined in many care homes. The frequency with which these categories of information were mentioned in the nursing notes was then recorded.

The nursing notes are a means of communication from one shift to the next, as well as a legal statement of what the nurse observed and thought was important. So it is reasonable to assume that if one type of information is recorded frequently, that this information is thought to be important.

See if you can guess what the nursing notes in the research reported most frequently, in order. Perhaps you would first like to guess where pain assessments were ranked (1-9), then put the others in order.

 Exercise 3

> **Place numbers from 1 to 9 beside each category, 1 being the most frequently mentioned and 9 the least mentioned:**
>
> *Category*   *Relative frequency*
>
> **Behaviour**
> **No change (care plan followed)**
> **Bowels/bladder**
> **Hygiene/ bathing**
> **Medical interventions**
> **Mobility**
> **Nutrition/feeding**
> **Pain**
> **Social (e.g. visit from family)**

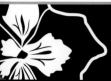

The answers from the nursing notes study are given below. In particular see where the category of pain assessment came in the scale of importance, and see how accurately you guessed.

Category	Relative frequency
Behaviour	2
No change (care plan followed)	1
Bowels/bladder	7
Hygiene/ bathing	9
Medical interventions	3
Mobility	4
Nutrition/feeding	8
Pain	6
Social (e.g. visit from family)	5

This gives us some idea of the fact that pain in a care home resident does not impact as strongly on nurses as some other experiences or behaviour of the residents. There may be legal or administrative reasons for this. However, to the older person who is in pain the reasons may seem unimportant compared to the fact that they are in pain.

e) Myths about Pain in Older People

 Exercise 4

Which of the following are true or false? *True/False*

1 Older people do not feel pain as much as younger people.
2 Older people do not worry about pain, since they are used to it.
3 Pain is part of growing older - you have to expect pain in old age.
4 There's not much you can do for pain in old age.

They are all false.

Fred went to the doctor complaining of a painful left foot. The doctor examined his left foot and leg. He could not come to a diagnosis as to the cause of the pain in Fred's foot. So the doctor said: "Fred, it's just old age" "Well" said Fred. "How is it that my right foot is not painful when it is the same age as the painful left one?"

What do you think Fred was saying to the doctor?

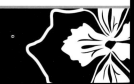

f) Attitudes of Older People towards Pain

Think of what could happen to you if you went to the doctor about a pain in the abdomen.

 Exercise 5

Write down the things that could possibly occur:

1   What might the doctor's attitude be?

2   What might the doctor do to you in his surgery?

3   What might he arrange to have done to you?

4   What might he prescribe?

5   What may happen to you if you took medication?

6   Is there a possibility that you may be fearful?

As you can see there are very real possibilities of unpleasant things happening if a person reports pain to the medical staff.

Many older people in care homes have these fears. Studies among older people living in the community have shown a lack of knowledge about pain management. They have also revealed attitudes that would hinder adequate pain management. Similarly, surveys of people living in institutional care have shown various reasons why older people do not report pain to their carers.

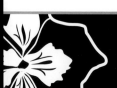

These include:

- Fear of painful investigation
- Denial - "If I ignore the pain it may go away"
- "I don't want to lose control in making decisions about my own body"
- "I don't want to bother other people"
- "I don't want to be thought of as a complainer"
- "I may be given drugs that will make me an addict"

One study in 1990 of 148 patients indicated that 10% of patients rarely complained because they thought it was a sign of weakness. Eleven percent viewed suffering as a challenge with positive effects; 13% perceived the pain as a punishment for some wrong deed.

NF12

All these factors may be present among older people in care homes. Even with early dementia a person may still have these ideas. If there has been a traumatic event with the medical profession in early life, this fear may persist or reawaken as the recent memory fails. Paranoia can also be part of the dementing process, and may add to the resistance to admit to symptoms.

g) Incorrect Staff Information and Attitude

Staff attitudes and knowledge are other factors preventing adequate pain management in care homes as well as acute care settings. Nurses and doctors sometimes have the attitude that older people have to expect pain. They can be overly concerned about dependency and addiction to medications. Imagine a casual or humorous remark by a nurse to the effect: "You don't want to take too much of that drug or you'll become addicted". This may give the wrong message to an older person who is already apprehensive about pain treatment. More and more evidence is accumulating that the use of narcotic analgesics prescribed for chronic non-malignant pain in older people has very little risk of causing dependence or addiction. Certainly, in the person with malignant pain and a limited prognosis, withholding adequate analgesia is ethically unsound. In the USA there has been successful litigation brought against a care home and the medical attendants because analgesic medication was withheld from an older man dying with prostate cancer.

NF13

Current good practice is to give regular doses of pain relief. However, some doctors still prescribe what is called PRN[1] ("as required") use of pain relief, although some residents might think it meant "Pain Relief Never". Forgetting simple measures such as heat packs, positioning and massage can mean that an older person is not as comfortable as possible, when pain is present from musculo-skeletal conditions.

Nurses should also remember that there is research which shows that the very presence of a caring nurse in close proximity to a patient leads to a significant reduction in perceived pain intensity, even though the nurse does not administer any treatment.

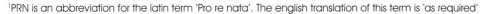

[1]PRN is an abbreviation for the latin term 'Pro re nata'. The english translation of this term is 'as required'

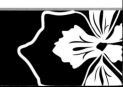

h) Loss of Control

When a person is a admitted to an acute hospital or to long-term care, he or she experiences two important changes as far as pain management is concerned.

1. There is loss of control. No longer can the person go to the medicine chest and take an analgesic tablet when in pain. In order to obtain medication there must first be communication with a nurse. Perhaps even some sort of negotiation will be necessary. The nurse may be too busy; the wait may be too long; the answer may be: "The doctor hasn't prescribed anything for you."

NF14

2. A new set of "significant others" enters the older person's world. Whereas a husband or a daughter may have been the carer and the one who related to the older person, now there are numerous nurses/support workers, some female and some male. This may present a threatening situation, especially if the memory and reasoning are failing. The attitudes of these new significant others can help or hinder the person expressing the need for pain relief. The nurse/support worker must in their verbal and body language give the very clear message of acceptance and understanding and readiness to care and respond to the person's needs.

i) Summary

This chapter has addressed the following topics:

- Older people living in the community have a significant prevalence of pain, especially in the joints, limbs and back.

- The most common disease causing this is arthritis.

- In acute wards, older people, especially those with dementia, do not receive analgesia as readily as younger more cognitive patients.

- In care home settings there is a high prevalence of pain among those residents who can respond verbally.

- Those with dementia receive less pain management than those with normal cognition. The reasons for this lie partly in the attitudes of the older residents and their ability to communicate their needs.

- The awareness, attitudes and knowledge of the attendant staff are also important in determining that pain is minimised among these vulnerable older people.

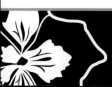

3 Knowing When Someone with Dementia is in Pain

Aim: To examine and reflect on the information available about pain assessment in people with dementia.

Contents

a) General Principles of Assessment

The process of pain assessment is one of communication. The professional communicates to the patient that he/she wants to know about the patient's experience. The patient then attempts to communicate this experience. It is important for the professional and the patient to feel comfortable in the assessment situation. If there is unnecessary tension, communication becomes distorted. The body language of the professional is most important in reducing any tension and in encouraging the patient to tell the story of the pain.

NF1

There is evidence that even though understanding of words is impaired or lost in more advanced dementia, people with cognitive impairment still remain sensitive to the tone of voice, the stance, the body movements and the facial expression of other people. So it is useful to remember this in trying to obtain a history of pain. If a person with dementia is disturbed by the staff members approach, their tone of voice or impatient attitude, the person with dementia will have increased difficulty in communicating about pain. It has to be realised that the person with pain is already stressed and another stress is even more difficult to cope with when their memory and emotional control are not working well.

A doctor standing at the end of the bed with arms folded and a frown on the face, speaking in a loud voice (because the patient/resident is hard of hearing and there is a lot of noise in the environment) is not the ideal situation for good pain assessment.

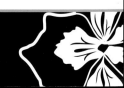

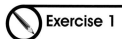

Exercise 1

Write down a list of simple things that could be done to help communication in the situation of a professional attempting to obtain a good history from an older person who is hard of hearing.

NF2

The professional wants to obtain the following information about the pain:
When it started; its site, nature, and intensity; and what are the exacerbating and relieving factors. Questions related to these aspects may need to be woven into a conversation and patiently unravelled from the communication.

The person with dementia's body language is also important in the communication. Just as the person is sensitive to the body language of the professional, the professional should be consciously attempting to observe and analyse the body language and facial expression of the patient.

b) Early Stage of Dementia

In a person with mild dementia the principles of pain assessment are very much the same as those for a person with no memory problems. The patient may have difficulty remembering information about the history of the pain. For this, the professional may need to rely on the help of a close relative or non-professional carer. Even this is not very different from what frequently happens in assessing a person with normal cognition. Information from the "significant other" is often an important source of history.

With all older people, but particularly those with early dementia, it is important to give the person time to respond to questions. Sometimes an older person will take 20 or 30 seconds to respond. The questioner may think that the person did not hear or did not understand or has forgotten the question. Patience is necessary.

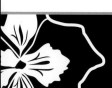

The Use of Pain Intensity Instruments

Some research has been undertaken to find out the usefulness of pain intensity instruments (such as visual analogue scales [VAS] or pain thermometers). There are difficulties in the use of various types of VAS with older people, especially those with dementia.

Visual Analogue Scale (VAS):
Please mark on the line how severe your pain is. 0 represents no pain at all, and 10 represents the most severe pain that you could have:

0   1   2   3   4   5   6   7   8   9   10

The person may have visual and/or hearing impairments that affect their understanding of the instructions; the older person may have difficulty using a pencil to mark a scale; cognitive impairment may prevent understanding the concepts of a VAS. However, despite these, it has been found that people with early dementia can often accurately indicate the intensity of their pain on a VAS. Modifications that may help are a vertical scale, rather than horizontal, the use of a yellow background, rather than black and white configuration. One successful VAS used with patients with dementia had the numbers 1 to 10 and, below the scale, an increasingly vivid colour scale progressing from pale pink under the number 1, through to vivid red at the end indicating most painful.

NF3

Another scale uses simple diagrams of faces with expressions varying from contentment to pain and asks the person to indicate which fits his/her pain the best. This may be an alternative if a VAS can not be completed. In using VAS or other pain intensity measurement, it will be necessary to give ample verbal instruction to the patient, and to allow for the possibility that there will be no instrument that can be completed.

The quickest was is to ask: "If zero is no pain and 10 is the most severe pain possible, on a scale of zero to ten where does your pain lie?" These scales only attempt to measure pain intensity which although important is only one quality of the pain experience.

In research conducted by the author, the most successful rating which included intensity was a simple question: "Is the pain a big problem, a medium problem or a small problem?" There were 151 people in pain in the care homes surveyed. Of these, 78 had mild or moderate dementia. Only two, who answered "Yes" to the question: "Do you have any pain at the moment?" were not able to give an answer to the question about the size of the problem.

c) Moderate Stage of Dementia

As cognitive decline continues, the ability to accurately describe pain becomes impaired, and carers cannot rely as readily on what the resident of the care home is telling about their pain. The nurse/support worker must look for other sources of information about the person's pain.

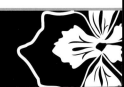

Sometimes a number of conflicting situations can arise:

1. Some older people are said to hide their deteriorating ability to perform, by making excuses about pain. This suspicion is very hard to prove because, as has been said in an earlier section, the only expert on a person's pain is the person. Others have pain that is hard to explain and to treat.

 Exercise 2

> Mr B was a 76 year old retired labourer, with no history of back pain before he presented in acute distress on five or six occasions to his general practitioner with overwhelming symptoms, screaming, shouting and crying uncontrollably. His ageing wife was unable to pacify him on these occasions and he had a number of admissions to hospital, where he was thoroughly investigated by the orthopaedic team. No cause for his pain could be found. He was referred to the geriatrician who once again could find no cause for the pain. Although Mr B was able to speak, his language was not fluent and his history was often inconsistent. One had the impression that Mr B was unable to cope with a pain problem, which in earlier times he could have tolerated. Eventually in discussion with his wife and daughter a decision was made to introduce increasing narcotics to try to relieve the pain. Narcotic analgesics were prescribed, as well as other medications, giving some relief, but his general condition deteriorated and he died. At post mortem he had evidence of pneumonia as a cause of death, but careful examination of the back structures did not reveal any disease process that could account for his symptoms.
>
> ***Do you think he had real pain? What was the correct clinical management of this man?***

NF4

2. In contrast there are cases in the literature where people with dementia and disease processes, which are known to be very painful, do not experience any discomfort. One recent case report is of a woman who had experienced severe chronic pain syndrome for many years, and who had attended a specialist pain clinic with very little improvement over many years. Her case was well documented. When she developed mild dementia, her complaints of pain disappeared. Even when questioned specifically about pain she denied any symptoms.

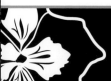

There is some evidence that as the brain becomes more affected by the process of Alzheimer's disease, the pain threshold is not affected, but the ability to tolerate acute pain increases if it continues. This means that if a person with dementia is being turned in bed, and this process is painful, the pain will still be experienced during the turning, even though more prolonged discomfort may not be registered in the behaviour or language. Thus if analgesic medication is prescribed, it should be given in anticipation of the painful procedure, to diminish the pain. This is not an excuse for under-treating the pain of people with dementia.

Another important consequence of the increased pain tolerance with cognitive impairment is that the person may tolerate pressure discomfort for so long that tissue damage and ulceration of pressure points may occur. So it is important to have very careful nursing when people with dementia are confined to bed.

d) Advanced Stage of Dementia

The important difference between moderate and severe dementia is the ability to communicate verbally. It is obvious that dividing dementia into three stages is artificial. The disease progression is inevitable but one particular ability can be lost in one person while being retained in another at about the same stage. However, eventually verbal expression becomes blunted and confused in most people with severe dementia. When this occurs, making a diagnosis of pain becomes a problem.

 Exercise 3

> One definition of pain is: "Pain is whatever the patient says it is." Think of this question: How can you be sure someone is in pain if they cannot tell you?

This question has challenged researchers and doctors. The research on this question has taken two forms:

1. There have been a few studies that set up situations in which people with dementia are subjected to essential pain (such as in receiving routine injections). The reactions of the subjects with normal cognition, and with mild dementia are compared with the reaction of those with severe dementia and no verbal communication. The assumption in some of these studies is that if the reactions are similar, then the reactions are to pain and can be used as an indication of pain in other situations. This seems a reasonable assumption.

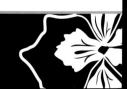

One problem is that this type of research can only be done ethically with acute pain. Why is this a problem? Write down what you think.

NF7

2. The second line of research attempts to extract from experienced practising nurses the strategies they use for making a diagnosis of pain in the person with advanced dementia. One assumption here is that nurses working on a daily basis in care home settings encounter the situation frequently and through this experience they acquire skills. Some of these skills can be analysed and handed on to others.

A number of studies have given us information on how nurses make a diagnosis of pain in non-verbal cognitively impaired patients. However, more research is needed to expand this field, and make it more valid and reliable.

e) Current Practice of Pain Assessment in Advanced Dementia

The practice of nurses in the field involves the use of observation of the person with dementia, as well as placing their observations in a framework that uses some reasoning or strategies. We will address these two separately, although expert nurses do not tend to separate them in practice.

1. **Observations:** For convenience, the observations can be placed into one of three groups:
      1.1 Physiological Changes
      1.2 Body Language Changes
      1.3 Behavioural Changes

1.1 Physiological Changes

Observation	
Change in colour	Change in pulse rate
Change in blood pressure	Change in temperature
Loss of appetite/fluid intake	Change of respiratory rate
Urinary/faecal incontinence	Change of sleep pattern
Sweating	Guarding

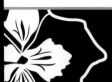

1.2 Behavioural Changes

Observation	
Aggression	Increased movement
Agitation	Decresed movement
Reaction to touch	Not weight bearing
Weeping/moaning	Increased confusion
Shouting	Hard to settle

1.3 Changes in Body Language

Observation	
Facial expression	Withdrawal
Assumes foetal position	Knee(s) drawn up

It will be seen that these classifications overlap somewhat. Behaviour and body language are hard to separate.

 Exercise 5

> When nurses are asked about their assessment of non-verbal patients they frequently say that they as practitioners 'just know' or have 'intuition' about the situation.
>
> What do you think these nurses mean when they speak of 'intuition' or 'instinct'?

NF8

One theory of learning proposes that becoming an expert in a particular skill involves the ability to move from following a set of rules to seeing the situation as a whole and being able to respond appropriately. One development in becoming an 'expert' is to be able to make 'graded qualitative distinctions'. This means being able to detect slight changes in a subject, such as change of skin colour, or change in tone of voice. In the assessment of a person who cannot speak, nurses make these graded qualitative distinctions. Nurses probably call some of these 'intuition'. For instance the ability to detect changes in ease of settling to sleep, or increased movement or changes in facial expression would be in this category.

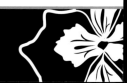

Facial Expression

One of the observations which is given importance in the assessment process is that of the facial expression of the person. Facial expression has been studied closely by psychologists, and a structured system called Facial Action Coding System (FACS) has been developed. This system divides the face into groups of muscles that move together In response to certain emotions to give facial expression. The FACS has not been devised using older people, nor people with dementia. Thus, using it to assess facial expression in dementia has been criticised. However, one research study used video clips and compared FACS with the opinions of ten practising nurses on whether people with dementia were expressing pain. The nurses' opinions agreed quite closely with the more complicated FACS.

One system for assessing 'discomfort' in non-verbal patients worked out by Dr Hurley in the USA is called the Discomfort Score for Dementia of Alzheimer's Type (DS-DAT). Although it is not specifically assessing pain, but rather discomfort from such things as fever, it has been modified and used in pain assessment. It contains items that depend on observations of both facial expression and body language, and involve graded qualitative distinctions.
For example, these items are:
- Looking sad
- Absence of a look of contentment
- Looking tense

So the present 'state of the art', is that change in facial expression is a useful way of diagnosing pain in the non-verbal person, especially in conjunction with other body language. However it must be remembered that more research needs to be carried out to more fully validate facial expression.

Pacing

One interesting piece of research has examined people with dementia who have lost their verbal communication skills and are physically mobile. The result of this study suggested that the presence of pacing as a chronic behaviour may be a sign of absence of pain, and an indication of reasonable physical health. However changes in physical movement, such as increased walking, may be an indication of the person experiencing pain. This should therefore inform the assessment process

f) Approaches to Pain Assessment

History of Pain Reaction

When a person with dementia is admitted to a care home, it is important to obtain from the carers what sort of reactions he or she had to pain in the past, as well as the types of activities that evoked pain reactions. This information should be recorded and reviewed when pain is suspected. As the older person lives in the institution any observations that are made which indicate reaction to pain should be recorded and shared among the staff.

NF8

Individual Personal Knowledge of the Person

Nurses and support workers rate this as the most important source of information, since this is what enables them to make these graded qualitative distinctions.

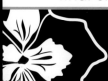

Disease Context

A maxim which experienced staff use is: "If a person without dementia has pain from a certain disease, then a person with dementia will have pain too". For instance, this means that the suspicion of pain is heightened if there is a diagnosis of rheumatoid arthritis or cancer in the bones.

Process of Elimination

If a change in behaviour is observed, which could be due to more than one problem, the member of staff should try to eliminate other causes, such as constipation or urinary infection. If these are not present, it is assumed that pain is present.

Validation by Assess-Treat-Reassess

This logical process is widely used by expert nurses. A resident has a change in behaviour etc. that could be due to pain. The assumption is made that pain is present. Treatment is provided, and the person is reassessed to see if the previous change has been reversed.

Repeat Observations by Multiple Observers

A new observer is asked to assess the patient/resident and the conclusions are compared. This discussion between staff is an important part of the process of pain assessment.

The Concept of Probability

It can be said that making a diagnosis is about probability. For instance, a person with central chest pain has a probability of having coronary artery disease; however it is not a certainty. If the patient is a 65 year old male, the probability is increased of having the diagnosis. If the patient is a 22 year old woman, it is less. When the 65 year old man is examined by his doctor after taking a careful history, there may be an increased probability. The result of an electrocardiogram may also increase the probability of a diagnosis being present. An exercise stress test will increase the certainty of the diagnosis. A coronary angiogram will make the diagnosis even more secure; in fact the probability of coronary artery disease may be sure enough for the expenditure of large amounts of money to operate on the coronary arteries.

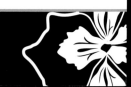

The process is one of increasing probability of a diagnosis being present. This same process is applied to making a diagnosis of pain. One can never be 100% sure, but a level of certainty can be attained for reasonable action to be taken.

Imagine Mr Robinson, an elderly man with dementia who cannot respond verbally. He has a diagnosis of Rheumatoid Arthritis, involving the hands, feet, elbows and shoulders. How sure are you that he has chronic pain? 100%, 90%, 80%, 75%, 50%, 25%, 0%.

If you guessed at 100%, you would be very brave. There are some people who have Rheumatoid Arthritis who do not have pain. Let us say that you guessed at 75%. This is the same as saying: "The probability that he has chronic pain is 75% or 0.75".

He is bed-bound, with contracture of the knees. He cannot feed himself, and cannot turn over in bed. When he is turned in bed by the nurses, he has facial grimacing and he withdraws his arms if they are touched. What is the probability of Mr Robinson having chronic pain? 100%, 90%, 80%, 75%, 50%, 25%, 0%. You may have increased the probability to 80% or 0.8.

You now provided him with some strong analgesic twenty minutes before the turning, and he did not grimace, nor withdraw when being turned. What now would be your estimate of the probability of pain in Mr. Robinson? 100%, 90%, 80%, 75%, 50%, 25%, 0%.

You may now be prepared to increase your probability estimate to 90% or even 100%.

This process was relatively straightforward in Mr Robinson's case. However the same process can be applied to more difficult diagnoses. If this process is followed and documented, it presents increasingly firm evidence for the nurse to present to the medical office in advocating for the person with dementia to receive good pain management.

Practical Results of Research into Pain Assessment in People with Dementia and Poor Language

The strength of the evidence that underlies the practice of pain assessment of the person with dementia and poor language has been published in 2002 in an important article written by the AGS (American Geriatrics Society)[1] . It looked at the evidence for the reliability of the observations that practitioners use in making a diagnosis of pain in the person with advanced dementia and poor language skills. The writers of this article concluded that there were six different areas that should be observed and recorded in making a diagnosis of pain in these

---

[1] AGS Panel on Persistent Pain in Older Persons. (2002) The management of persistent pain in older persons. *Journal of the American Geriatrics Society, 50* (6 Supplement), S205-S224.

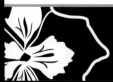

circumstances. Observations of some or all of these areas are included in various tools that are available for assessing pain in people with poor language. Some tools are useful for everyday use in busy settings; others are too cumbersome and are more useful for research purposes.

The six areas that may be observed are:
1. Facial expression
2. Negative vocalisation
3. Body Language
4. Changes in activity patterns or routines
5. Changes in interpersonal interactions
6. Mental status changes

A useful website is cityofhope.org. On this website there is a section which compares ten tools for assessing pain in non-communicating people with advanced dementia. These tools have been developed over the years 1992-2004. They are:

- The Abbey Pain Scale (Abbey J, et al., 2004)[2]
- ADD: The Assessment of Discomfort in Dementia Protocol (Kovach CR, et al., 1999)
- CNPI: Checklist for Non-verbal Pain Indicators, (Feldt K., 2000)
- Doloplus-2 (Wary, B and the Doloplus Group 2001)
- DS-DAT: Discomfort Scale-Dementia of the Alzheimers Type (Hurley A et al., 1992)
- FLACC: The Face, Legs, Activity, Cry and Consolability Pain Assessment Tool (Merkel SI et al., 1997)
- NOPPAIN: Nursing Assistant-Administered Instrument to Assess Pain in Demented Individuals (Snow AL et al., 2001)
- PACSLAC: The Pain Assessment Scale for Seniors with Severe Dementia (Fuchs-Lacelle SK et al., 2004)
- PADE: Pain Assessment for the Demented Elderly (Villaneuva MR et al., 2003)
- PAINAD: The Pain Assessment in Advanced Dementia Scale (Warden V et al., 2003)

The content of the observations of these tools is summarised in Table 1. For instance, the tools that sample all six areas recommended by the AGS are the Abbey, ADD and FLACC, however the FLACC has been developed for infants and has not been tested on elderly, demented subjects. The Abbey scale also includes a section on physical changes associated with pain,

[2]Abbey, J. A., Piller, N., DeBellis, A., Esterman, A., Parker, D., Giles, L., Lowcay, B. (2004). The Abbey Pain Scale. A 1-minute numerical indicator for people with late-stage dementia. *International Journal of Palliative Nursing, 10*(1), 6-13.

Kovach, C. R., Weissman, D. E., Griffie, J., Matson, S., & Muchka, S. (1999). Assessment and treatment of discomfort for people with late-stage dementia. *Journal of Pain & Symptom Management.*, 18(6), 412-419.

Feldt, K. S. (2000). The Checklist of Nonverbal Pain Indicators (CNPI). *Pain Management Nursing*, 1(1), 13-21.

Doloplus Group Website. http://www.doloplus.com

Hurley, A. C., Volicer, B. J., Hanrahan, P. A., Houde, S., & Volicer, L. (1992). Assessment of discomfort in advanced Alzheimer patients. *Research in Nursing& Health, 15*(5), 369-377.

Merkel, S. I., Voepel-Lewis, T., Shayevitz, J. R., & Malviya, S. (1997). Practice applications of research. The FLACC: a behavioral scale for scoring postoperative pain in young children. *Pediatric Nursing, 23*(3), 293-297.

Snow , A.L., Hovanec, L., Passano, J., Brandt, J. (2001). Development of a pain assessment instrument for use with severely demented patients. Poster session presented at the Annual Meeting of the American Psychological Association. Washington, DC.

Fuchs-Lacelle, S., & Hadjistavropoulos, T. (2004). Development and preliminary validation of the Pain Assessment Checklist for Seniors with Limited Ability to Communicate (PACSLAC). *Pain Management Nursing, 5*(2).

Villanueva, M. R., Smith, T. L., Erickson, J. S., Lee, A. C., & Singer, C. M. (2003). Pain assessment for the dementing elderly (PADE): Relaibility and validity of a new measure. *Journal of the American Medical Directors Association* (Jan/Feb), 1-8.

Warden, V., Hurley, A. C., & Volicer, L. (2003). Development and psychometric evaluation of the pain assessment in advanced dementia (PAINAD) scale. *Journal of the American Medical Directors Association*(Jan/Feb), 9-15.

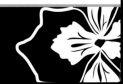

such as skin tears, pressure areas, arthritis and contractures, so it goes beyond the non-verbal communication to include other data in making the diagnosis of pain.

The rigour of the testing of the tools during their development is also an issue and this has been addressed by the City of Hope group. The DS-DAT, the PACSLAC and ADD scored best on the criteria used to address this evaluation of the tools. It should be noted that the ADD is more than a tool for assessing pain but is a protocol with interventions to develop a treatment plan." This is desirable, but means that it is attempting more than the other tools with which it is compared.

Having a tool to use in assessing a person's pain is only the start. The next thing is to learn to use the tool properly. Some of the tools mentioned above are quite complete and involve observations of all six areas recommended by the AGS group; others do not address all these areas for informing about the presence of pain. However some require significant amounts of training in order to be reliable. Others involve more time than is available in a busy aged care facility. So in choosing a tool it is important to consider who is going to do the assessment and where the tool is to be used. Perhaps the Abbey Pain scale is the most practical of these tools and can be used with relatively little extra training. The assessment of pain may only take a few minutes. A copy of the Abbey pain scale has been included as appendix A in this booklet by kind permission of Professor Jennifer Abbey.

Table 1

AGS Guidelines	Abbey	ADD	CNPI	DS-DAT	Doloplus2	FLACC	NOPPAIN	PADE	PAINAD	PACSLAC
Facial Expression	+	+	+	+	+	+	+	+	+	+
Vocalisation	+	+	+	+	+	+	+	+	+	+
Body Movements	+	+	+	+	+	+	+	+	+	+
Changes in interpersonal interactions	+	+	+			+				
Changes in activity patterns and routines	+	+	+			+	+			
Mental status changes	+	+				+				

g) Summary

In this session we have looked at the way that pain is diagnosed as the dementia progresses, stressing that the verbal responses of the person with dementia must be listened to and acted upon, in the same way as those of a person with normal cognition.

When dementia becomes advanced and verbal communication becomes impaired, the diagnosis is made using observations of physiological changes, body language (especially facial expression) and behavioural change. These are interpreted by the experienced member of staff in the context of certain logical processes. The process is one of increasing probability of the diagnosis being correct.

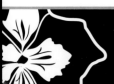

4 Ideas Into Action

Aims: To consider some of the ethical issues in relation to pain management.
   To consider some principles of treatment of pain.
   To apply the ideas of the previous sessions to practice.

Contents

a) Some ethical issues
b) The importance and use of a diagnosis - responding
c) The importance and use of a diagnosis - advocating
d) The importance and use of a diagnosis - aspects of treatment
e) Revision: making an assessment of pain
f) Revision: making an assessment of pain well enough to be an advocate
g) The culture of an institution

a) Some Ethical Principles

- Maximising Personal Control
- Enabling Choice
- Respecting Dignity

These are principles of good dementia care but they are not always easy to apply in practice. They are illustrated below using individuals so you can take your own view on them.

Maximising Personal Control

 Exercise 1

> Consider the following situation:
>
> Fred was 78 years old. He had been in a care home for two years, admitted because of dementia. His wife had died and no family could care for him prior to admission. He was unsafe with domestic appliances, had tended to walk on the roads, and was a danger to himself and others. He also had arthritis in the hips. Fred has had a severe bleed from the stomach because of arthritis tablets and it is considered that he should not have this type of medication. Fred's habit was to walk along the hallways and out into the sheltered garden whenever he could for long periods. During the winter months Fred's arthritis became worse and on the days that he walked in the garden it was noted that he complained of pain in the legs. Despite repeated explanations regarding the link between his pains and his walking in the cold, Fred continued to attempt to get outside in the garden in the cold.
>
> What should be done about this?

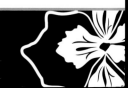

Enabling Choice

Exercise 2

Consider the staff response

After staff discussion about Fred's problem, the decision was made to give Fred the choice each time he wished to go out into the cold. Since he could not readily remember the consequences of his actions, the staff strategy was to remind him of the link between the pains and the cold garden walks, and ask Fred to make a choice each time. It was also decided to encourage Fred to put on extra warm clothing before going out, and to get a warm pack on Fred's hips as soon as he came in from the garden. All went well until the snow came. Fred wanted to go for his walk in the garden. A young nurse was in the process of getting his warm clothes for Fred, when a senior nurse decided that it was too cold for walking even though the snow was only a few inches thick. Fred was forbidden to leave the building. He was most agitated.

What should be done about this?

Respecting Dignity

Exercise 3

The following is the story of Grace.

Please read the story and write down what you think about the maintenance of Grace's dignity in the situation.

Grace was 83 years old. She had been a newspaper reporter in her youth and middle age, and had achieved the position of editor of an important newspaper before entering management at the age of 55 years. She became quite wealthy. At the age of 79 years, Grace developed dementia. She was admitted to an exclusive private care home where she was cared for very well. Her ability to make decisions about her own health and care was very limited. She then developed cancer of the stomach. She was experiencing abdominal pain and loss of appetite. Her family asked for a referral to an eminent surgeon, working privately, who had great success with this disease. After consultation, the surgeon was of the opinion that he could give her a 50/50 chance of survival if he operated using a new technique that involved complex prolonged surgery and a number of follow-up procedures over a period of twelve months. Grace would have to have various tubes in place for this time to keep her nutrition adequate. Initially she would be in a private hospital for probably three months having this treatment, then in another institution for more nursing care than could be provided in the private care home where she had settled. The family asked what the alternative was. The answer was given "To give her morphine and let her die."

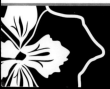

Grace, as you will have recognised, presents a very major ethical dilemma. Should she receive very expensive, complicated and potentially very confusing surgery to relieve her pain (and possibly cure her) or should she be given pain relief and be allowed to die? You might like to talk to your colleagues about this.

There is no right answer but there are a lot of useful questions that help in these situations such as:

- What are the views of each of her family?
- What are the views of each doctor, nurse and care assistant?
- What might her views have been?
- What decision might have been made if she was 33 not 83?

b) The importance and use of a diagnosis - responding

The challenge of making a diagnosis of pain in a person who is unable to use language is not only found in caring for people with dementia. It is also an issue in addressing the needs of some people with a developmental disability or who have had a stroke, causing aphasia. In all these circumstances one must think about how to respond to the patient's needs. As has been mentioned before, the pain needs of these people are often neglected by health providers. The motivation for the author writing this booklet is to help professionals address the needs of these people.

c) The importance and use of a diagnosis - advocating

Not all doctors, nurses or support workers are sensitive to the needs of these people, and it may be necessary for an individual practitioner to advocate to other professionals or even to family carers on behalf of the person with poor language. Sometimes the professional staff members have to negotiate with a guardian or the family to obtain relief for the person.

Many people with advanced dementia who cannot speak are in the terminal phases of the condition. It is important to remember that dementia is a fatal condition and that many people in the terminal phase are in pain because of their inability to get into comfortable positions, or because of fixed flexion deformities of the joints. Some professional carers may not recognise this and may need to be convinced that a response to the persons' pain is necessary, and that the principles of palliative care should be in place.
The scope of this book does allow for us to look in detail at advocating but there is an article that may be helpful.[1]

---

[1] McClean WJ (2003)Pain in clients with dementia: advocacy, ethics and treatment: Nursing & Residential Care 5 (10) 481- 483.

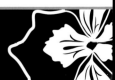

The principles are:
1. Be well prepared with information
2. Work out clearly what you think the person needs
3. Understand the emotional needs of those to whom you are advocating, such as the doctor or other nursing staff or family
4. If at first you don't succeed, try again

d) The importance and use of a diagnosis - aspects of treatment

There are various modes of providing comfort for the older person and these can be grouped into two approaches. They should be used together.
1. Non-pharmacological treatment
2. Analgesic Medication

1. Non-pharmacological treatment
It is wise before treating a person with medication to ask: "Is there another way of treating the pain that does not involve medication?" Most analgesics have the potential for side-effects that can be unpleasant, so if they can be avoided that is better.

Here is a list of Non-pharmacological modes of pain treatment. You may be able to add to the list:

Positioning
Massage
Heat or Cold
Reassurance
Distraction
Supporting a limb
Mobilising

2. Analgesic Medication
There are certain principles of pain treatment that are important in the older person. These are:
• Keep the number of medications to a minimum. Try to manage with a single analgesic, rather than a mixture.
• Give the medication regularly for chronic pain. "PRN" medication generally does not provide good pain relief.
• Opioids are not contraindicated for chronic pain, especially in older people where other modes of treatment, such as surgery, are not possible.
• Drug "addiction" is a rare phenomenon in the older person who is being treated for chronic pain.

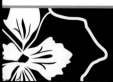

One of the issues that staff face when caring for people with dementia is that the person will not take medication when their discomfort is obvious and the pain is disturbing their life experience. One should consider the use of alternative routes of drug administration:

- Liquid medications may be appropriate if the person dislikes/has difficulty swallowing tablets.
- Trans-dermal "patches". Some opioid analgesics are available in this form. If a person with dementia have difficulty swallowing or accepting oral medication a patch is sometimes a useful way of providing relief.
- Regular subcutaneous morphine may be very helpful in the terminal phases and the use of a syringe driver makes the relief more certain.

e) Revision: Making an Assessment of Pain

 Exercise 4

Alex was a 77 year old man with advanced dementia. He had been in a care home for two years. Over this time he had been very active. From early morning until early evening he would be found walking around the home. He was very thin, but ate well and rarely demonstrated behaviours that challenge. He had only confused words which rarely made sense. One morning the staff nurses noted that Alex was still in bed. He was not interested in moving from a flat position. If a nurse attempted to raise him to sitting position he would pull away. His temperature was slightly elevated (37.8o C), pulse was 110/min.

Using the following checklist answer the following questions:

What would you be looking for in assessing Alex?

Outline what further process you might undertake to assess Alex?

Usual behaviour	Probability of pain =
Observation	Probability of pain =
Vital signs	Probability of pain =
Facial expression	Probability of pain =
Behavioural change	Probability of pain =

How probable it is that Alex has pain?

How could you increase the probability of your diagnosis being correct?

Alternatively try to use the Abbey pain scale to make the diagnosis, and see if you come to the same conclusions.

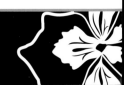

f) Revision: Making an Assessment of Pain well enough to be an Advocate

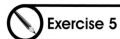 **Exercise 5**

Edna was a 95 year old great-great-grandmother who had severe dementia. She was bedbound and unable to feed herself. She was doubly incontinent and had no verbal communication. Each day her two daughters (both in their mid 70s) visited Edna. As Edna deteriorated she commenced non-specific verbalisation with high-pitched screaming, which would go on for some time after any disturbance, such as hygiene after incontinence. Edna was not prescribed any medications. The doctor responsible for Edna's care was known to not favour giving medication to patients with dementia. Discussion with Edna's daughters indicated that they felt this to be a sign of pain, since that was how they remembered their mother reacting when she had a kidney stone some years previously.

The other people in the same ward as Edna complained about the noise. One resident said: "She should be thrown out of the home for making such a racket!" On a number of occasions Edna's blood pressure was measured while she was crying out, and it had risen from her usual 130/85 to 190/90, and her pulse had risen from 80/min to 110/min. After a week of the doctor refusing to contemplate any change in Edna's medication, a meeting of the nursing staff was held. Three of the most experienced nurses had examined Edna while she was crying out, and they felt that her facial appearance expressed pain. One of the staff was elected to gather together the data to advocate to the doctor on Edna's behalf to obtain analgesic medication for the presumed pain.

You are the one elected to gather the data. Using the following form, write in what you are going to say to the doctor.

Using the following checklist attempt to state how probable it is that Edna has pain?

Usual behaviour	Probability of pain =
Observation	Probability of pain =
Vital signs	Probability of pain =
Facial expression	Probability of pain =
Behavioural change	Probability of pain =

History of previous pain behaviour	Probability of pain =
Association between activities and behaviour	Probability of pain =
Staff "conference"	Probability of pain =

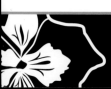

Use the Abbey Pain scale to confirm the diagnosis.

 Exercise 5 continued

Family concerns:

Dignity issues:

 Exercise 7

Using this data try to compose the message that you would convey to the doctor in advocating for Edna.

g) The Culture of an Institution

Each individual staff member helps to create what can be called the "culture" of the institution where older people live. This culture will place priorities on various activities and roles. One facility may pride itself in the beauty of the gardens and the furniture and fabric of the buildings. Another may place emphasis on cleanliness. Still another may have the culture that efficiency is the prime aim.

 Exercise 8

Think about the following event:

A doctor had been attending a patient in a care home. The doctor felt that the patient had some pain, but was not admitting to the symptoms. After the consultation he met the senior nurse whom he had known for many years. He had first worked with her as charge sister of the coronary care unit in the local hospital. He had great respect for her as a person and as a nurse.

He asked this nurse: "Christine, how many residents in the nursing home do you think are in pain?" Christine answered: "I don't think any are in pain. We look after these people with tender loving care."

What do you think about the culture of this nursing home with respect to pain management?

Is it enough for the staff to treat each resident with "tender loving care"? Or should there be an awareness that a certain percentage of the residents may be in pain and that these should be sought out and their pain addressed? How can the culture of the facility be changed to have increased awareness of the need for pain management?

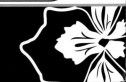

h) Summary

In this last section we have attempted to draw together some of the ideas that we have been dealing with in the other three sections, and apply them to situations that are found in care homes or other institutional care. We have seen that decisions involving people with dementia should be made within the value framework of principles which are involved in maintaining the personhood of the one who has dementia. The day-by-day decision making is not always simple. The issues of risk-taking and enabling choice are often in conflict. These same issues are involved in pain management.

We have also looked at some issues and actions that ensue after a diagnosis and assessment of pain have been made in a person with very poor language skills.

The further development of the skills of pain assessment by staff working with people with dementia will be enhanced by careful observation and documentation, as well as the sharing among colleagues of the knowledge and ideas that arise in good clinical practice.

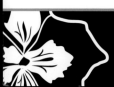

Chapter 5 – Notes for Facilitators

Introduction: The practice guide is designed to enable a facilitator to develop a series of individual education sessions or a study day. The individual exercises along with the 'Notes for Facilitators' are set out to be used to guide staff through the stages of engaging with the issues of pain in older people and people with dementia. The notes below provide additional information to a facilitator who is providing education on pain management to a group of staff.

The facilitator can reproduce these materials for use in an education session, but must reference any materials reproduced to the source materials. Copyright is only granted within this context.

Notes for Facilitator Chapter 1 - What is the Problem?

NF1

Attempts to define "pain" are helpful to highlight the fact that pain is a subjective experience. It is a very personal event. Try to lead the participants to see that it is:
a) Personal/subjective; b) Unpleasant; c) Difficult to define; d) May have a meaning for the person who is suffering.

NF 2

In this session the aim is to be achieved by commencing with experience that is common to humans - the experience of pain. We then try to move the participants from this common experience to appreciate some of the peculiar issues that people in institutional care deal with as they experience pain. Some of the issues can be appreciated by imagining situations to which we can all relate. So the story of George is a starting point. Thinking about George's experience should help the participants to appreciate the three elements of pain experience as found in the given definition of pain.

NF 3

The idea is that the pain George was experiencing is not worrying him, because he associates it with the pleasant gardening that he did the previous day. Thus the knowledge of the gardening and the pleasant emotions were colouring the pain experience to neutralise at least some of its unpleasant nature.

NF 4

The knowledge/emotions that George had are now being doubted by George because his previous experience of similar aches tells him that they should have worn off by now.

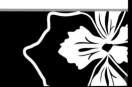

Once again the knowledge has changed the emotion and the significance of the pain has changed; hence its nature.

The knowledge about George's pain has now changed. There is a sinister element to the pains, although the intensity of the sensation apparently has not changed. The knowledge change has led to an emotional change, and the significance of the pain is now different.

As well as long–term memories from childhood impacting on the pain experience the person may not be able to reason that particular pain is NOT threatening. They may then react more violently than we would think appropriate. The clinical significance of this is that the person with dementia may need to be reassured before a painful procedure, such as an injection. There is evidence that people with dementia do not see the clues that a painful situation is about to occur (such as a nurse approaching with a needle and syringe); the reaction to the painful stimulus is therefore greater than in a person who cognitively anticipates the pain.

This exercise reinforces the issues addressed regarding the three aspects of pain. Athletes' motivation is based on knowledge of the outcome they desire - to win or to achieve a personal best, or even to finish the course! This puts the pain in the context of sensation, knowledge and emotion.

Different schemes of pain classification are used for different purposes. One scheme used to try to analyse the cause of pain classifies the sensation into:
"Nociceptive", where the sensation is able to be explained by the degree of activity of the peripheral neurons. The nervous system is believed to be intact.
"Neuropathic", where the pain is thought to be due to damage of the nervous system.
"Idiopathic", where the pain persists in the absence of identifiable organic disease.

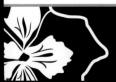

Burning a finger on a hot iron	A
Osteoarthritis of the knee	CN
Heart attack (myocardial infarction)	A
Peritonitis from perforated stomach ulcer	A
Cancer of the breast involving the vertebrae	CM
Osteoporotic fractures of the spine	A but can become CN
Pain after an attack of shingles	CN

Although these definitions are a little technical, staff will probably have met them or will come across them. It is useful to stress that pain threshold is not the only aspect of pain which can be measured formally or even informally. One hears clinicians talk about a patient as having a "low pain threshold". Often the term is used wrongly. It may be worth while discussing this with the participants, especially in terms of attitudes towards patients. The "low pain threshold" is often used in a derogatory way when speaking about patients.

Experienced staff will have stories to tell of their experience of different people's pain expression. It may be helpful to let the participants share some of these experiences. It will be important to try to stay neutral in relating these, and to point out that the mode of expression is culturally influenced. There is research evidence of these differences, though we should not stereotype too rigidly. For those participants working in older age care it is important to bear in mind that differences may exist between generations in the use of language about pain.

The participants may like to explore the reasons why underestimated pain is commonly found. This does occur in care homes and acute cancer wards. The assessment of both nurses and medical staff showed no correlation with the patients' visual analogue scores (VAS) of pain intensity apart from those patients who recorded very little or no pain.

Possible explanations that should be explored are:
a) Denial by staff members who, for emotional reasons, have problems dealing with the fact that the person is in pain.
b) Lack of personal experience of pain. (There is evidence that there is a greater correlation between the patient's VAS scores and the staff members' VAS scores where the staff member has a history of significant personal pain experience).

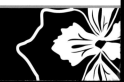

As well as an activity in the group, it may be worth while encouraging participants to do this exercise with some of their colleagues in the workplace and report back to the group at a later date, if the course is being run over a period of weeks.

It should be noted that the absence of these changes does not exclude the presence of pain. Of course, if these signs are present then they are significant.

Encourage the participants, from their own experience, to think of other examples of how body language can give a clue for the presence of pain.

The effects on close significant others should be highlighted. For those living in the community and interacting with family, chronic pain affects relationships, sometimes dramatically. Dependence, co-dependence and other unhelpful relationships may develop.

The other issue to explore is the way in which chronic pain in a resident in a care home affects the staff. Frustration can lead to difficulties; the possibility arises of conflict between staff members over the proper attitude towards the person with chronic pain complaints. The ideas on how to manage the person's needs may differ between staff members. (Some staff members may see a dependency relationship developing between the resident and one nurse, while that nurse sees the other members as unfeeling).

The matter of equity arises. How much time and attention can be allocated to one individual?

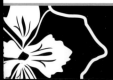

Notes for Facilitator Chapter 2 – Older people in Pain

NF1

Because most professionals live independently in the community, this session starts with elderly people's experience there. Thus participants are more likely to relate to that experience. It is hoped that this session will help the participants move emotionally to be more empathetic with the experience of living in residential aged care.

NF2

These studies, done in the USA, were mostly phone interviews. The participants could discuss whether there would be a difference in the prevalence of pain among older people living in their own country. Does phone interviewing obtain different responses compared to face-to-face techniques? There may be differences in the community's readiness to admit to pain. However the range of conditions causing pain should be similar.

NF3

There are factors in the patient such as:

Poor communication skills

Poor memory of how to get the attention of the nursing staff (e.g., bed-side call system)

There are factors in the staff such as:

Staff attitude towards pain

Staff time

Priorities of care

Inadequate medication protocols

Management attitudes

Staff ignorance

Poor handling techniques

Lack of physical therapist services

NF4

Participants may have experience of visiting or being in an acute ward. This may lead to useful discussion.

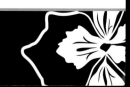

Factors which may affect the prevalence of pain in a care home will include:

- The prevalence of various diseases that may cause pain, especially arthritis.
- The communication skills of the residents.
- The knowledge of the staff.
- Staff attitudes about pain.
- Management's attitudes about pain.
- Medical officers' skills and attitudes regarding pain management.

These research details are given to show that the problem is one which has been studied and that the issue is important. The details are not to be remembered, but the general principle is of concern.

Participants need to understand that it is likely that 30% of their residents may be experiencing pain.

The purpose of this question is to make participants aware that a difference in perception exists between staff and residents.

Give the participants time to discuss their ranking of these categories, before providing the findings of the research. No doubt there will be some discussion as to the reasons for their choice. This is useful, since it focuses on the documentation habits and their relevance to the comfort of the residents.

Obviously the issue here is a doctor covering up his inability to come to a diagnosis, and taking refuge in a *myth* about ageing: that aged people should expect pain.

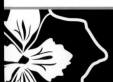

Write down the things that could possibly occur:
1. *What might the doctor's attitude be?* Unsympathetic; unbelieving of the level of pain; realistic and very active in pursuing the diagnosis.
2. *What might the doctor do to you in his surgery?* He may perform examination that is embarrassing or painful.
3. *What might he arrange to have done to you?* Tests such as X-rays or blood tests that may be painful and distressing.
4. *What might he prescribe?* Medication or surgery that may be unpleasant.
5. *What may happen to you if you took medication?* Side-effects may occur that are unpleasant.
6. *Is there a possibility that you may be fearful?* Yes. All these may make you fearful, as well as knowledge of the diagnosis which may not be pleasant.

These ideas could be explored with participants to find out if they had considered them as issues in their care of the older person/person with dementia.

This case brought by the family against the care home management and the medical officer involved, claimed after the man's death that his pain and suffering were unnecessary and preventable. Even in retrospect a large damages settlement was awarded to the man's estate. This may not happen as readily in other countries as in the USA, but the issues of morality, justice and equity - rather than money - are equally important.

An exercise, which may bring home this issue of control, is to have a role-play in which one of the participants acts as a patient and another acts as a nurse with poor attitude. A third could act as a charge nurse and a fourth as a doctor who is difficult to convince of the need for analgesia. The negotiation at these levels should help to reinforce the loss of control that the patient experiences, and the fact that the doctor is so distant from the patient's experience.

The participants should be encouraged to tell the story of someone that they care for professionally for whom they have become a "significant other". You could explore with them what signs there are that this relationship has been established.
- What things does the resident share with you?
- How do you feel about the resident?
- How does this differ from your feelings about other residents?
- What about your feelings when a resident dies?

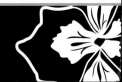

Notes for Facilitator Chapter 3 - Knowing when someone with dementia is in pain

NF1

An exercise which will demonstrate this is for the participants to break into pairs. One member of the pair will be asked to tell the other about something that greatly interests him/her. This may be a hobby or some experience that they have had. The other member of the pair is to continually shake her head and turn away, giving the partner the body language of discouragement.

Try to encourage the participants to say how they felt during the exercise.

NF2

The participants should be asked to write down what simple things could be done to encourage better communication in this situation. Suggestions:
- Take patient into a quiet room
- If possible get two chairs so that you can get close to the person
- Make sure that hearing aids are working
- Consider using a paper and pen if appropriate
- There may be one member of staff who is very good at communicating with that resident
- Family members may help

NF3

Some of the participants may have had experience of using Visual Analogue Scales with pain assessment in care homes. Try to sample their experience and share this with the group.

NF4

The answer must be that the man had pain, because "pain is whatever the patient says it is". The words "real pain" imply that there is such a thing as "imaginary pain". Such a concept is dangerous for professionals to entertain.

The intention of the orthopaedic surgeon, to discharge him from hospital to the care of his wife, was an abdication of professional responsibility.

The message from this story is that there are some extremely difficult problems to which there are no easy answers, but care and empathy must be provided. Communication with the family as well as the patient is very important in making decisions.

NF5

It should be stressed that these cases are so unusual that they are written up in the medical journals. The probability of any one of us meeting one of these cases is extremely small.

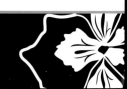

NF6

Any change in the abilities of a resident should stimulate the question: "Why has this person changed?" It could be a urinary infection, a fractured hip or constipation. Encourage the participants to explore these possibilities.

NF7

The issues are:
a) subjecting vulnerable people with dementia to chronic pain is not ethically acceptable;
b) the very nature of chronic pain means that the physiological and behavioural changes found in acute pain are not found in chronic pain.

NF8

It would be useful to ask the participants to discuss the assessment of a person, with dementia, who was previously peaceful, but develops a new behaviour of pacing. This may in fact indicate discomfort from constipation or pain from some other source.

NF9

In particular, experienced nurses do not hold an "all-or-nothing" understanding of verbal communication in patients with dementia. Often a nurse who knows her patient well can extract valuable information from the patient's "non-specific verbalisation". The participants should be encouraged to share experiences where this has occurred.

It is valuable to have knowledge of previous behaviour at a time when a diagnosis of pain was clear. Often this knowledge is not documented. Methods could be explored of documenting and raising staff awareness of significant behaviour.

NF10

The participants could discuss other painful conditions, and make a list of possibilities. It must be remembered that if a person has cancer it does not necessarily mean that there will be pain. About 40% of people dying from malignant disease will have pain.

NF11

The participants could discuss the question of change in behaviour due to constipation. Increased confusion and difficult behaviour can arise from constipation. Is this, in fact, an experience that should be classed as "pain"?

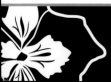

NF12

Validation by assess-treat-reassess:
This process is an important part of the assessment process. The participants could be encouraged to share experiences in which this process was used.

NF13

On the other hand, when more than one observer is involved, confusion can occur as a result of disagreement. Then the arbiter could be to apply the "validation by assess-treat-reassess" process. The process of repeating observations should include an agreed format, which we will introduce in the next session.

NF14

The purpose of introducing this concept is to show that the process of nurse diagnosis of pain is as intellectually respectable as medical diagnoses. The fact that one cannot be 100% sure is a fact of clinical life.

NF15

This (75%) would be a reasonable guess. It could be pointed out that just using this information means that the clinician could expect to be correct about 75 times out of 100 cases, and incorrect in the other 25 cases.

NF16

It should be noted that the extra information leads to increased probability of pain being present. Explore the other possibility, that, if there was no facial grimacing and no withdrawal, what happens to the post-test probability of pain? It leads to a reduction in the probability of pain, but not a probability of zero.

NF 17

Discuss with the participants the fact that they may be prepared to place more reliance on certain pieces of information than on others. The 'strength' of the information gives a greater difference between the pre- and post-test probability.

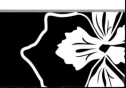

Notes for Facilitator Chapter 4 – Ideas into action

NF1

The issue is one of allowing control and allowing risk, while attempting to minimise the risk. There may be a number of responses to the situation, including applying hot packs, or a hot bath, as soon as Fred has finished his time outside. An outing to a warmer place for a walk may be a possibility. The participants may well have other solutions.

NF2

Sometimes the motivation for treatment is at best "mixed". In Grace's situation, one must suspect that the surgeon's desires for income or notoriety or practice of a new procedure were over-riding Grace's welfare.

NF3

The participants should realise that their role as advocates is fulfilling their duty of care to the resident or patient. Since people with dementia are disempowered they need someone with normal cognition and communication skills to take their part and advocate for them. The issue of pain management is only one area in which this advocacy is needed.

The participants could be encouraged to explore other issues in which their advocacy is needed for the people with dementia under their care.

One of the important points about successful advocating is that the information should be relevant and organised. It should be presented in a way that shows:
a) what was observed
b) what was the reasoning
c) what was the ultimate conclusion

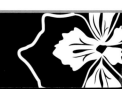

Appendix A

Abbey Pain Scale

For measurement of pain in people with dementia who cannot verbalise

How to use scale : While observing the resident, score questions 1 to 6.

Name of resident : ....

Name and designation of person completing the scale : ....

Date : .... Time : ....

Latest pain relief given was...at.........hrs.

Q1.   Vocalisation
eg whimpering, groaning, crying   Q1 [   ]
Absent 0   Mild 1   Moderate 2   Severe 3

Q2.   Facial expression
eg looking tense, frowning, grimacing, looking frightened   Q2 [   ]
Absent 0   Mild 1   Moderate 2   Severe 3

Q3.   Change in body language
eg fidgeting, rocking, guarding part of body, withdrawn   Q3 [   ]
Absent 0   Mild 1   Moderate 2   Severe 3

Q4.   Behavioural Change
eg increased confusion, refusing to eat, alteration in usual patterns   Q4 [   ]
Absent 0   Mild 1   Moderate 2   Severe 3

Q5.   Physiological change
eg temperature, pulse or blood pressure outside normal limits,
perspiring, flushing or pallor   Q5 [   ]
Absent 0   Mild 1   Moderate 2   Severe 3

Q6.   Physical changes
eg skin tears, pressure areas, arthritis, contractures,
previous injuries   Q6 [   ]
Absent 0   Mild 1   Moderate 2   Severe 3

Add scores for 1 - 6 and record here ⟹ Total Pain Score [   ]

Now tick the box that matches the
Total Pain Score ⟹

0 - 2	3 - 7	8 - 13	14 +
No pain	Mild	Moderate	Severe

Finally, tick the box which matches
the type of pain ⟹

Chronic	Acute	Acute on Chronic

Jennifer Abbey, Neil Piller, AnitaDe Bellis, Adrian Esterman, Deborah Parker, Lynne; Giles and Belinda Lowcay (2004) The Abbey pain scale: a 1-minute numerical indicator for people with end-stage dementia . *International Journal of Palliative Nursing*, Vol 10, No 1pp 6-13.
(This document may be reproduced with this acknowledgement retained)

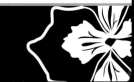

Use of the Abbey Pain Scale

The pain scale is best used as part of an overall pain management plan.

Objective

The pain scale is an instrument designed to assist in the assessment of pain in residents who are unable to clearly articulate their needs.

Ongoing assessment

The scale does not differentiate between distress and pain, therefore measuring the effectiveness of pain-relieving interventions is essential. Recent work by the Australian Pain Society[1,2] recommends that the Abbey Pain Scale be used as a movement-based assessment.

The staff recording the scale should, therefore, observe and record on the scale while the resident is being moved eg, during pressure area care, while showering etc.

Record results in the resident's notes. Include the time of completion of the scale, the score, staff member's signature and action taken in response to results of the assessment.

A second evaluation should be conducted 1 hour after the intervention taken in response to the first assessment, to determine the effectiveness of any pain relieving intervention.

If, at this assessment, the score on the pain scale is the same, or worse, undertake a comprehensive assessment of all facets of the resident's care, monitor closely over a 24 hour period, including any further interventions undertaken, and, if there is no improvement, notify the medical practitioner.

[1] Australian Pain Society(2005) Residential Aged Care Pain Management Guidelines, August.
http://www.apsoc.org.au

[2] Gibson, S., Scherer ,S and Goucke , R (2004) Final Report Australian Pain Society and the Australian Pain Relief Association Pain Management Guidelines for Residential Care: Stage 1Preliminary field-testing and preparations for implementation. November

Jenny Abbey
June 2006

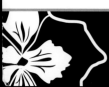

Further Reading

Australian Pain Society (2005) Residential Aged Care Pain Management Guidelines, August.
http://www.apsoc.org.au

City of Hope Pain & Palliative Care Resource Center
http://www.cityofhope.org/prc/elderly.asp

Faull C, Carter Y and Woof R. (1998) *Handbook of Palliative Care* Chp.9 Oxford: Blackwell Science

Fordham M and Dunn V (1994) *Alongside the person in pain* London: Baillière Tindall

Horn S and Munafo M (1997) *Pain: Theory, Research in intervention* London: Open University Press.

Kerr D, Cunningham C, Wilkinson H 2006. Responding to the pain experiences of older people with a learning difficulty and dementia
http://www.jrf.org.uk/bookshop/details.asp?pubID=784

Mccafferty M and Beebe A (1994) *Clinical Manual for Nursing Practice* London: Mosby

Mcquay H and Moore A (1998) *An Evidence-Based Source of Pain Relief* Oxford: Oxford University Press

Munafò M and Trim, J (2000) *Chronic Pain. A Handbook for Nurses* Oxford: Butterworth-Heinemann

National Council for Hospice and Specialist Palliative Care Services and Scottish Partnership Agency for Palliative Cancer Care (2000) *Positive Partnerships: Palliative Care for Adults with Severe Mental Health Problems* London: Department of Palliative Care and Policy

Royal College of Physicians/British Geriatrics Society/British Pain Society, (2007), The assessment of pain in older people

The Patients Association (2007), Pain in older People - A Hidden Problem
http://www.patients-association.org.uk/onlinewebmanager/downloads/Pain%20in%20Older%20People%20-%20A%20Hidden%20Problem.pdf

Quality Improvement Scotland (2006) Best Practice Guide: Management of chronic pain in adults.
www.nhshealthquality.org

Sign Guidelines (2000) *Control of Pain in Cancer Patients: A National Clinical Guideline* Edinburgh: Scottish Cancer Therapy Network

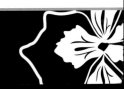